BLESSED BY BREAKFAST

RENÉE TARANTOWSKI BAUDE

Balboa Press books may be ordered through booksellers or by contacting:

Balboa Press
A Division of Hay House
1663 Liberty Drive
Bloomington, IN 47403
www.balboapress.com
1 (877) 407-4847

Because of the dynamic nature of the Internet, any web addresses or links contained in this book may have changed
since publication and may no longer be valid. The views expressed in this work are solely those of the author and do
not necessarily reflect the views of the publisher, and the publisher hereby disclaims any responsibility for them.

This book is a work of non-fiction. Unless otherwise noted, the author and the publisher make
no explicit guarantees as to the accuracy of the information contained in this book and in some
cases, names of people and places have been altered to protect their privacy.

ISBN: 978-1-9822-0503-4 (sc)
ISBN: 978-1-9822-0504-1 (e)

Print information available on the last page.

Balboa Press rev. date: 06/12/2018

BALBOA.
PRESS
A DIVISION OF HAY HOUSE

Dedication

To my beloveds, we are all walking each other home.
Especially my Daddy and Ken, 49 was too young for you to pass, I can feel your spirits guiding me each day.

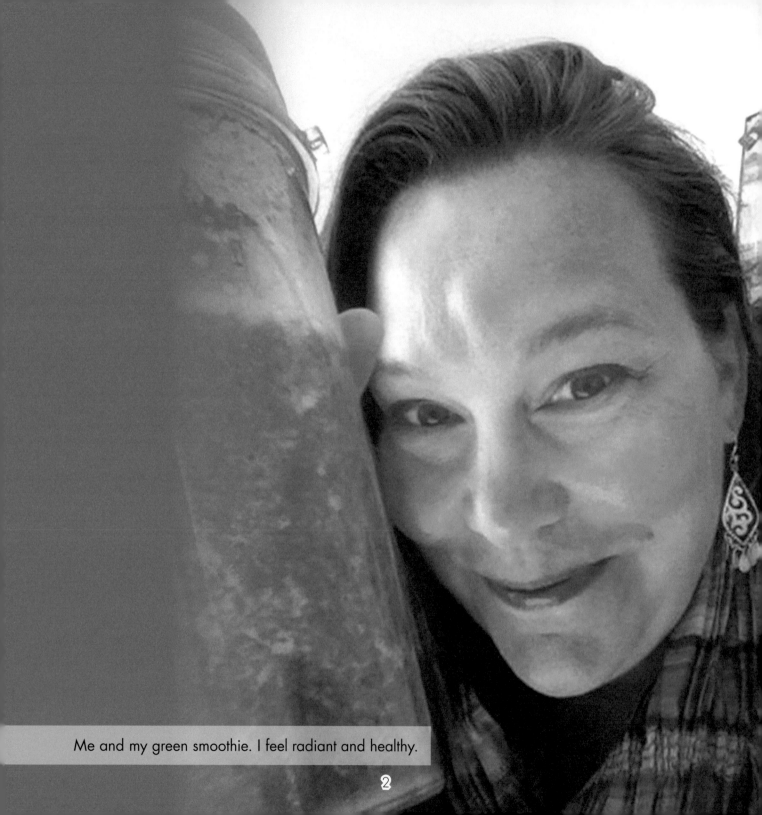

Me and my green smoothie. I feel radiant and healthy.

2

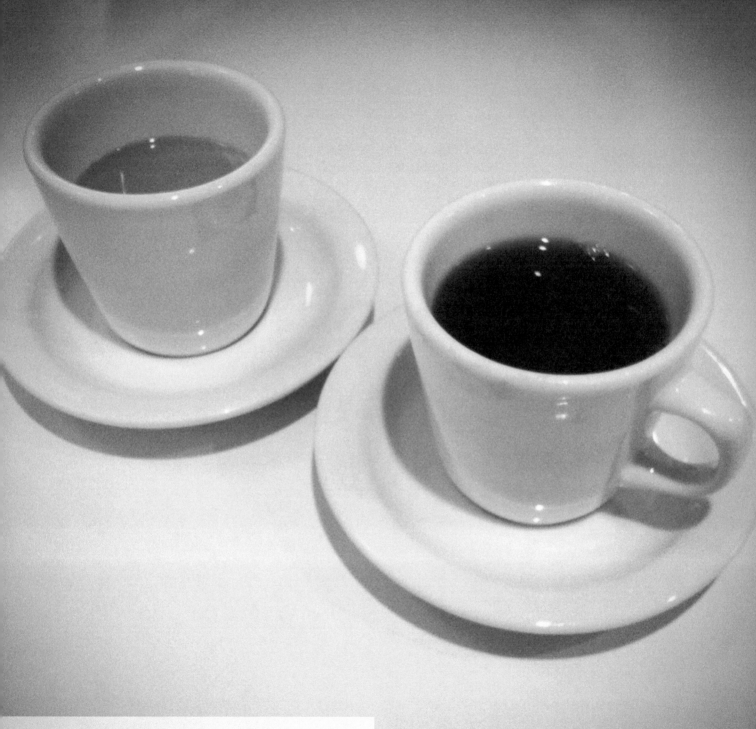

Coffee for two. I'm a hopeless romantic.

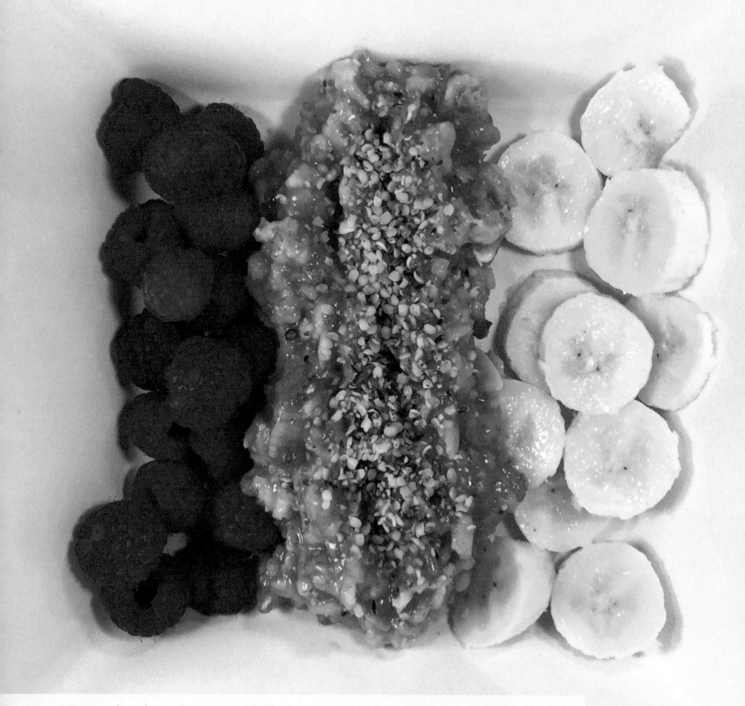

Roasted walnuts, bananas, blueberries, top oats, rice quinoa with hemp seeds

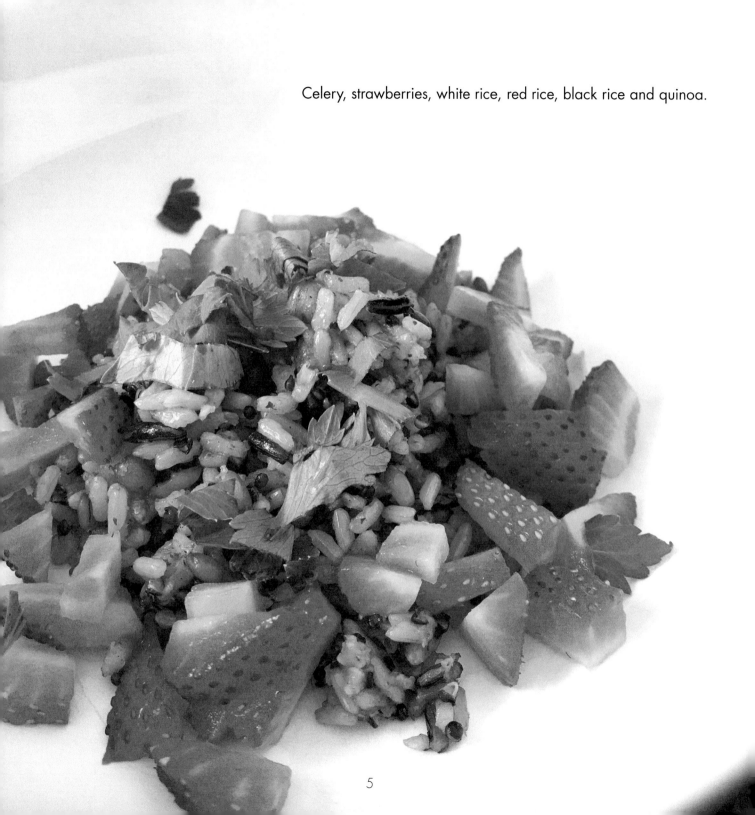

Celery, strawberries, white rice, red rice, black rice and quinoa.

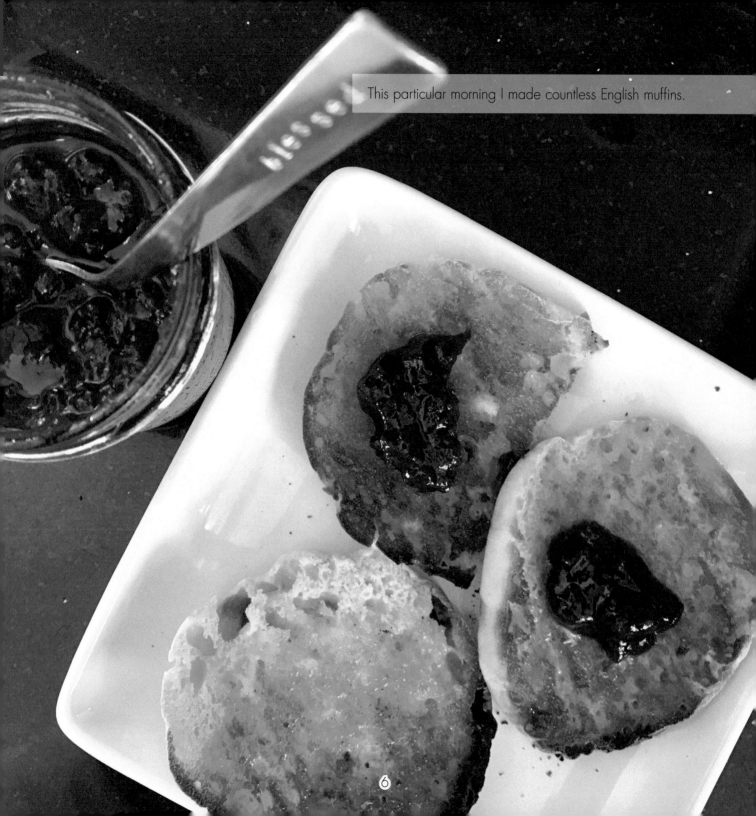

This particular morning I made countless English muffins.

Introduction

I have been writing the perfect cookbook for decades. I've pitched to publishers with rejections starting to equal the number of my recipes. I didn't get it. I was pitching the kind of cookbook I wanted to buy, the kind of cookbook that sprang from wonderful conversations with grandma-types at weddings, after church, funerals, and knitting circles. I'm a magnet for grandmas and recipes. I cook, I take photos, I write and make notes, and occasionally hit publish on my blog or Instagram. I do it for myself because food is sacred and life giving. The colors, textures, and smells make me feel alive, especially when I grow my own food. I also do it for my kids, my friends, and legacy. Not only my own legacy, but also the legacy of wise women walking this journey before me.

But all the food blogging and solitary kitchen time was recently disrupted. You see, I have had several friends "go vegan" for two weeks—just two weeks. Then, during those two weeks it all changed. I was their go-to vegan recipe writer. Their results have been remarkable. I'd also add that they are all over 50 years old! They feel amazing, look younger, feel younger, have lost the leg pain, and some have told me sex is better. (I am a vault, but they said I could tell you!) I'm not at all surprised they are feeling great.

Then, some of these same friends wanted their reluctant spouses and partners to try eating a plant-based diet. My standard answer was "go to my website and search around," but they didn't want to hunt and peck, they wanted a concise easy guide in their hands to use every day. So here we are. I started out writing this book for a few people, but I think everyone can benefit from the wisdom and mindfulness within the recipes. Coming together to sustain life—sharing a potato, a box of mac and cheese split between four people, or a feast—we come together to share our daily bread for richer or poorer—in community.

I've known my friend who asked me to write an article on vegan breakfasts, which started this whole vegan cookbook journey, since high school. I was thrilled she reached out and that I could help. I am honored to share in her community and I'm honored to also share in yours—we are all connected.

I wanted to write an amazing cookbook, but like so many things in my life, I find joy in doing and not in documenting. I've slowly been changing that. After years of head down grinding away at life, I'm changing my mindset to sharing and delighting in every conversation. I see now I am better served, and serve better by sharing, engaging, and listening. I'm thrilled to have you on this journey.

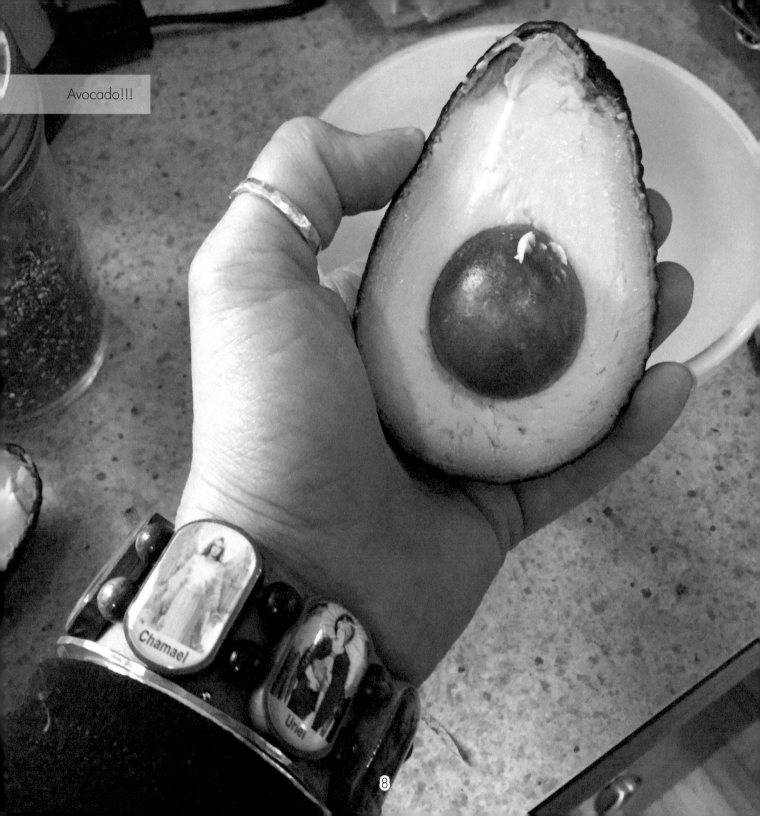

Avocado!!!

8

ESCH ROAD
EST 2012
ALL NATURAL
GREAT LAKES · TRUE FOODS
ON OUR FARM

Local bread with local jam. Does it get any better?

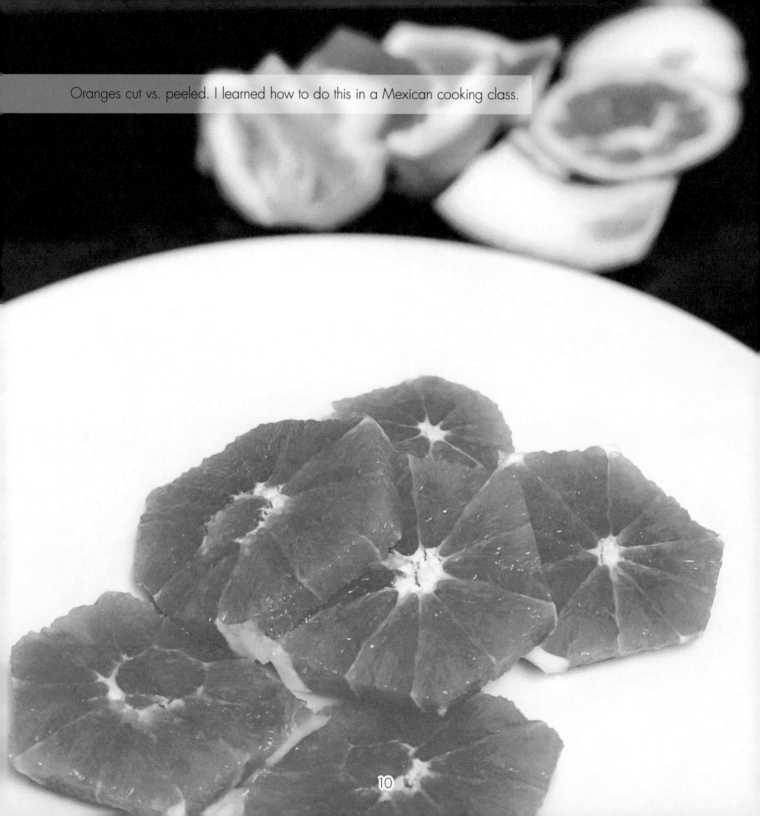

Oranges cut vs. peeled. I learned how to do this in a Mexican cooking class.

If eating mindfully is a goal, I invite you to follow along for inspiration, hand holding, and recipes—because we all need tons of support when we are starting something new, and not quite mainstream. This book also feeds my desire to be a Home Economics teacher and Mindfulness Guide so it's a win for everyone. I have learned from the best and I'm eager to share my simple ways of creating a sacred space at the dining room table. This book is so much more than food and photos. It is love, soulful, simple, sacred, beauty, and mindfulness.

Truth: I am blessed by breakfast because of the wonderful people (and one dog) I wake up with!

BREAKFAST TIME

Each new day gives us the opportunity to start over, and breakfast is the perfect time to launch into mindful eating and living. I intend to begin the day with love, light, tenderness, awareness, and respect. Somedays are better than others but setting my intention helps when I get off track. It isn't about how many times you fall off the wagon, it is how quickly you get back on that matters.

I have always enjoyed a very simple and cozy breakfast—coffee with toast, eating in bed with a newspaper. My family likes a little more variety so initially buying boxes and boxes of cereal made sense, until one day it no longer did. (Full disclosure: one of my kids loves cereal and I'm ok with that, I respect that choice.)

Many, many factors went into my decision to "ban the box" from our daily breakfast table. I didn't like the idea of giving my kids a "meal" of processed, sugary, limited nutritional value that left them hungry. Gradually, I began a morning practice of silently blessing my family with simple, nutritious, plant-based foods for breakfast. Muffins, fruit, oatmeal, and toast with yummy jams served with coffee or tea. Doesn't that sound divine!?!

After we banned the boxes from the breakfast table I needed to find a new way. To make breakfast interesting, plant-based, and not processed, I quickly came up with a rotation of several vegan morning treats to delight the senses and make my family feel great.

Breakfast is a meal that sets the tone for the day, and sometimes I want my day to start with as many options as possible; creamy, fluffy, warm, sweet, or savory. I set my intention:

I am blessed by breakfast because of . . . (each day I finish this sentence with tender words from my heart.)

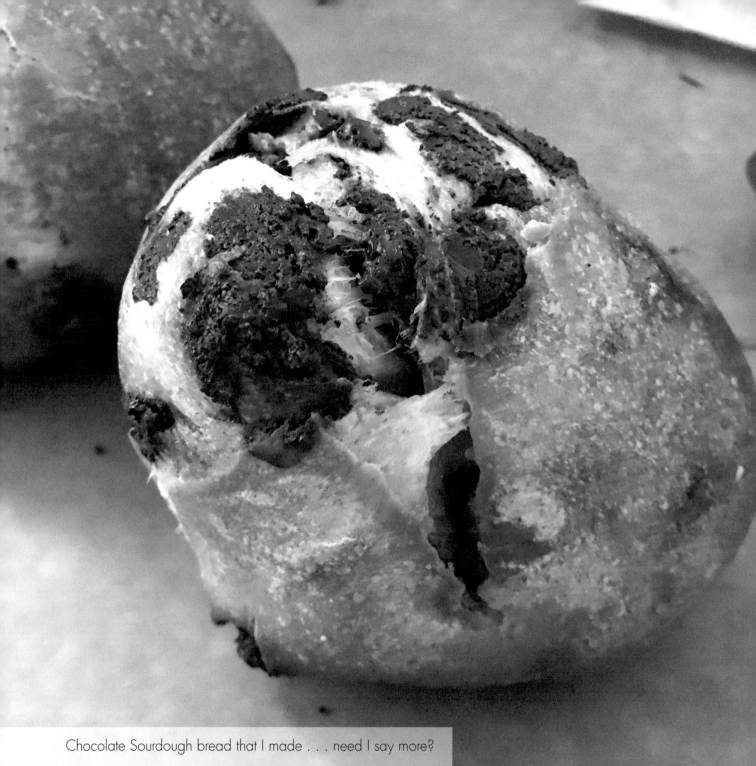

Chocolate Sourdough bread that I made . . . need I say more?

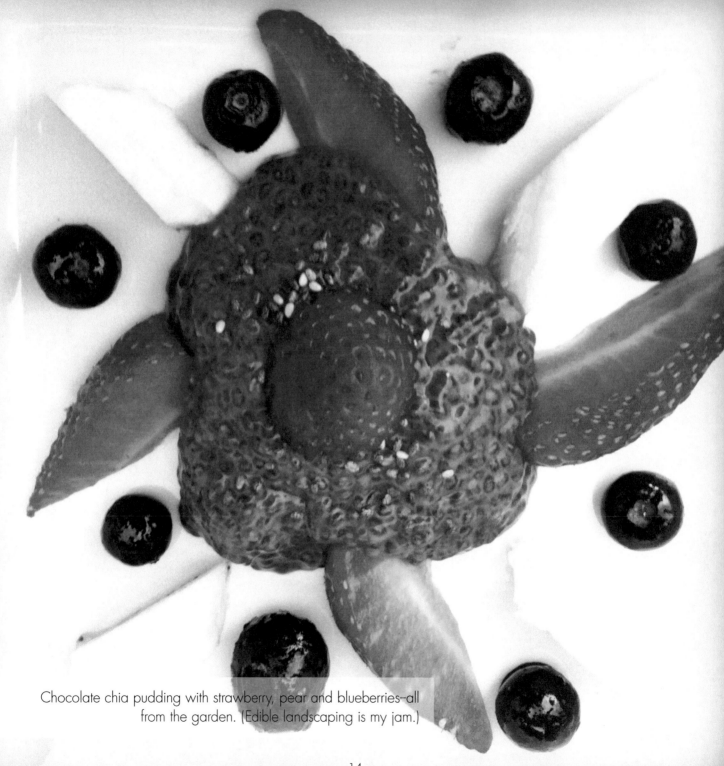

Chocolate chia pudding with strawberry, pear and blueberries–all
from the garden. (Edible landscaping is my jam.)

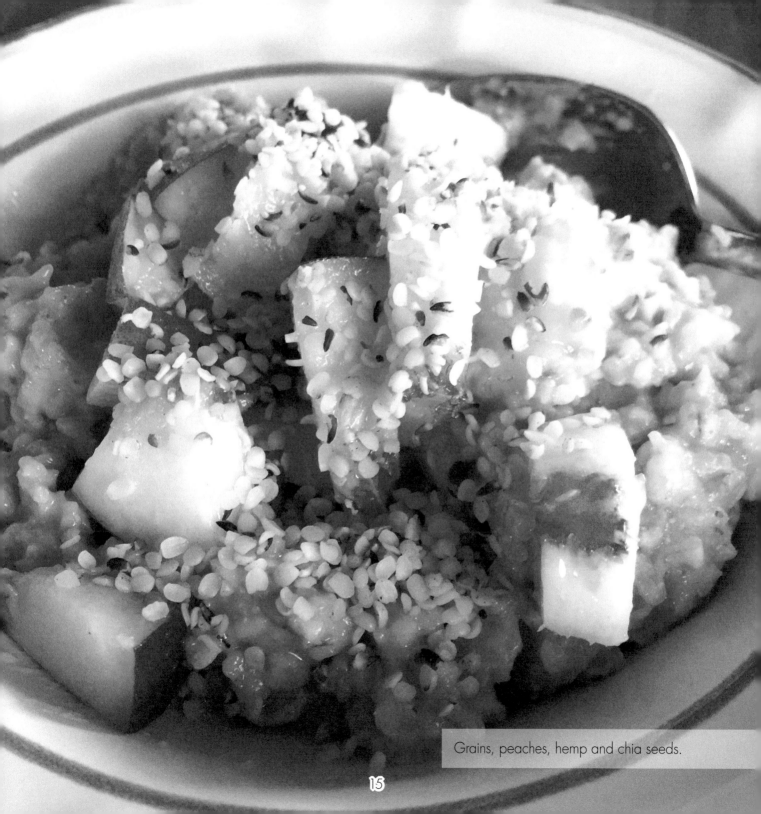

Grains, peaches, hemp and chia seeds.

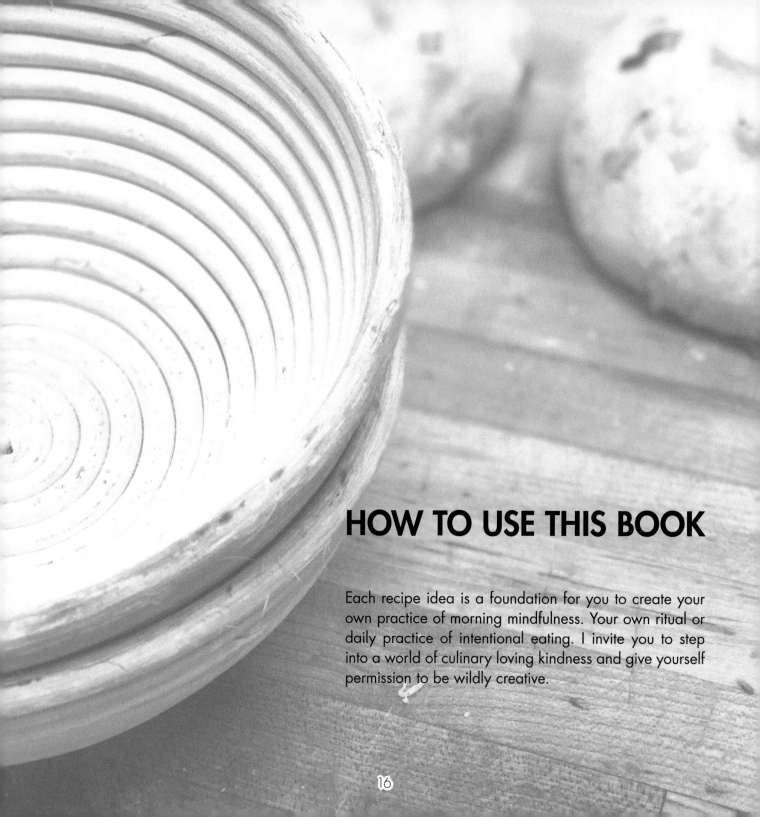

HOW TO USE THIS BOOK

Each recipe idea is a foundation for you to create your own practice of morning mindfulness. Your own ritual or daily practice of intentional eating. I invite you to step into a world of culinary loving kindness and give yourself permission to be wildly creative.

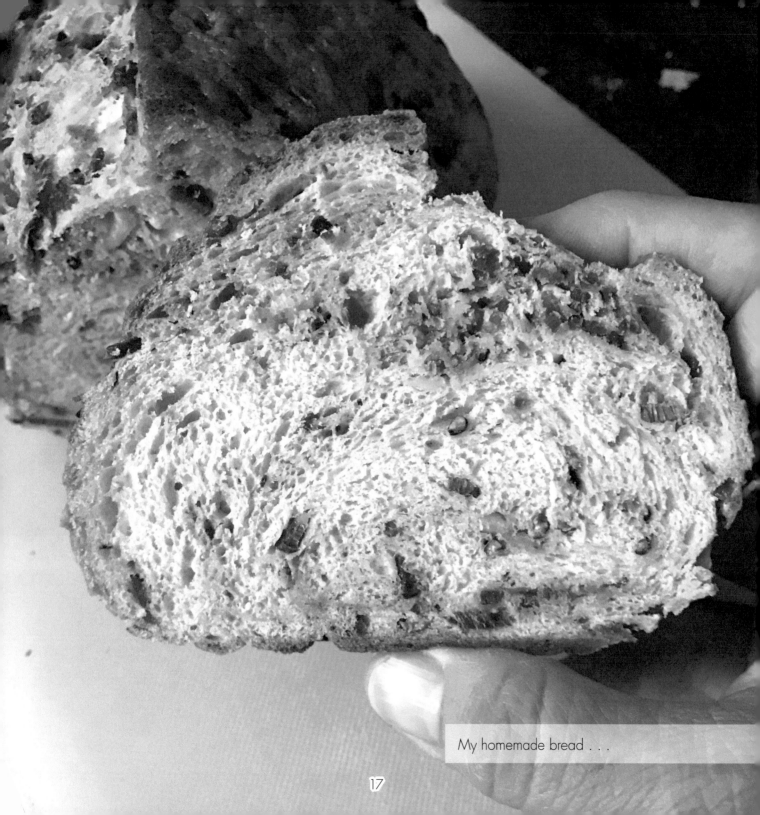

My homemade bread . . .

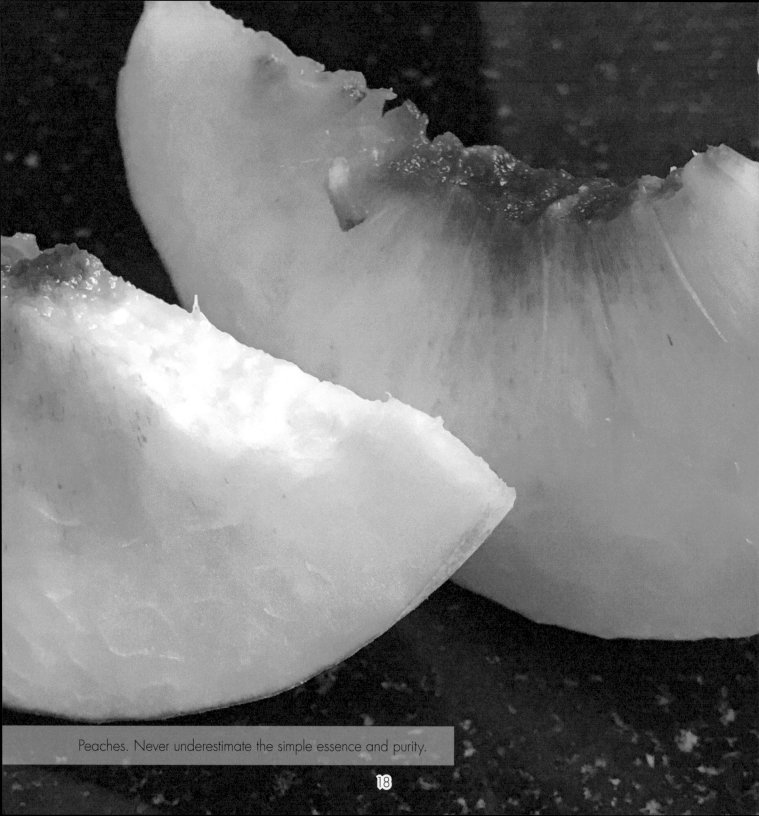

Peaches. Never underestimate the simple essence and purity.

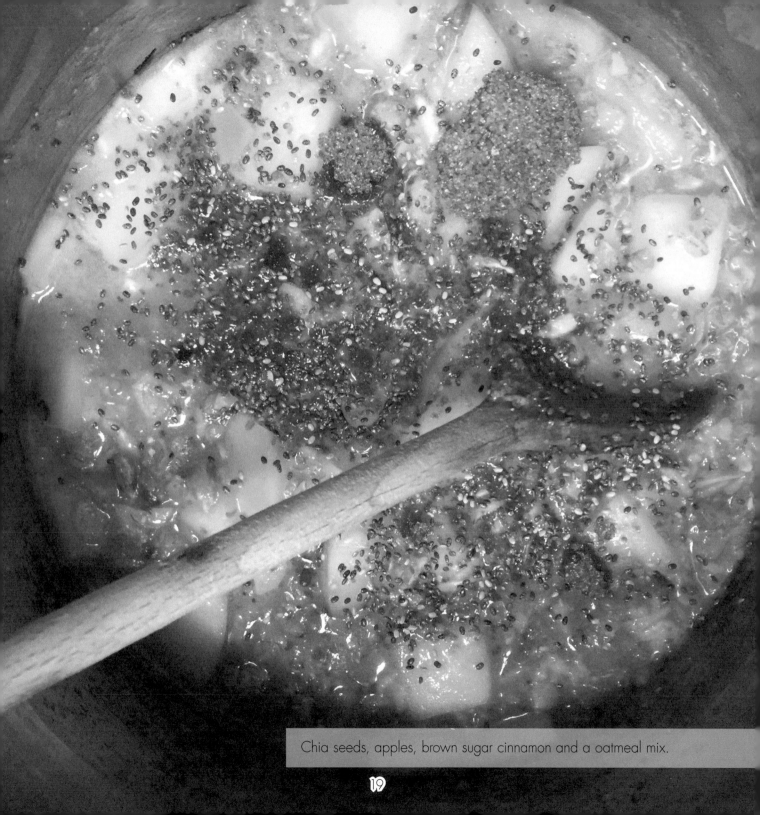

Chia seeds, apples, brown sugar cinnamon and a oatmeal mix.

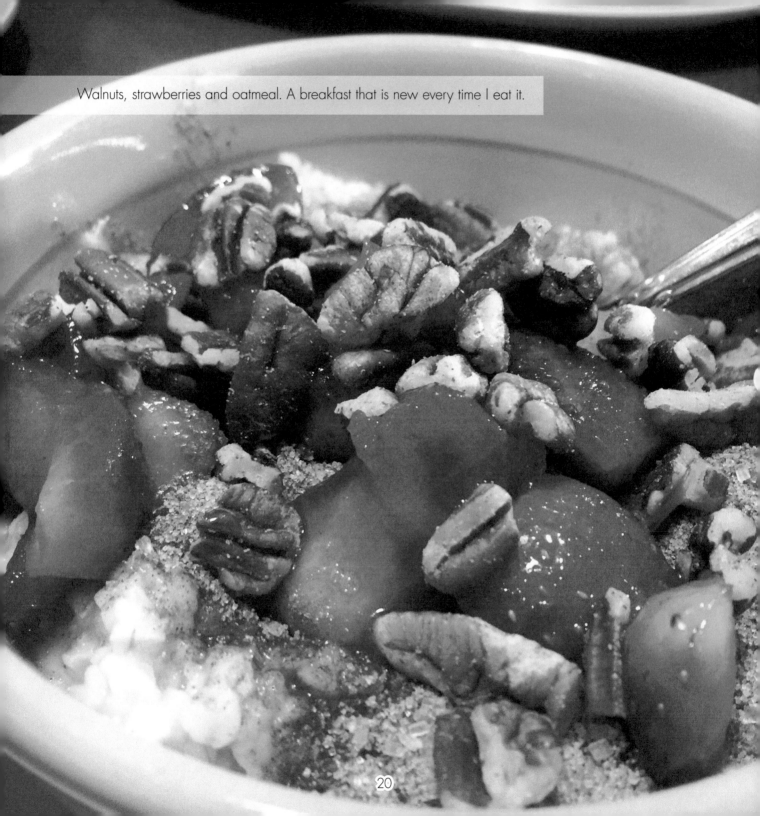

Walnuts, strawberries and oatmeal. A breakfast that is new every time I eat it.

Road tripping with a green drink and fuel for the road.

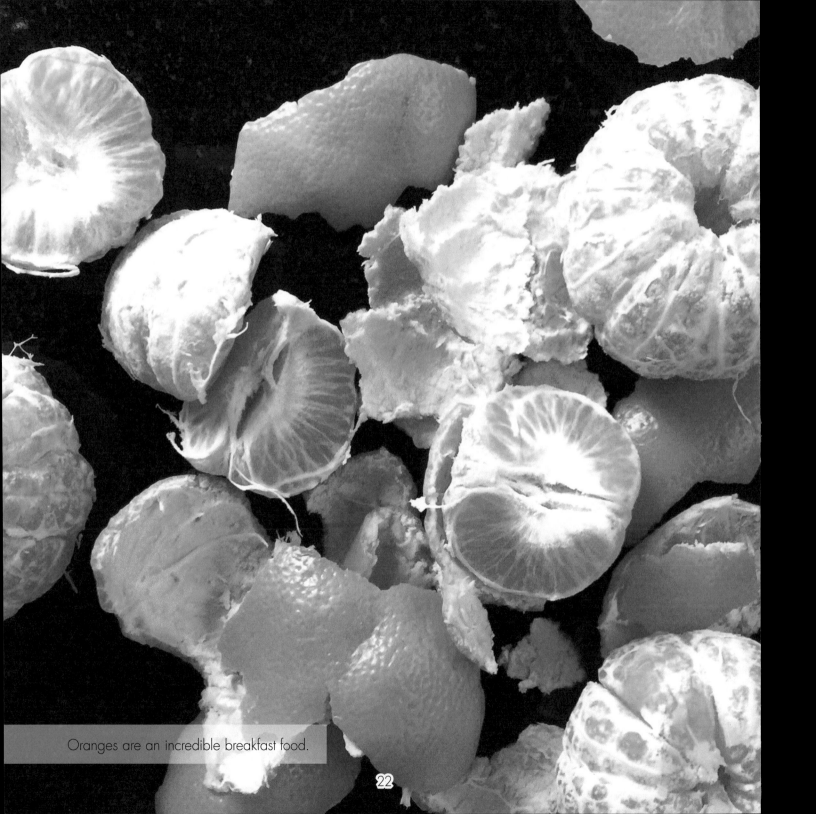

Oranges are an incredible breakfast food.

BREAKFAST 1: VEGAN TOAST

Toast is my go-to breakfast.

Let's be honest. Toast is not exactly a culinary challenge BUT when you think of toast as a blank canvas waiting for the artist to create from a place of love and mindfulness—it becomes an edible expression of our inner untapped creativity.

Coffee, toast with Earth Balance Spread and local jam. This works perfectly for those of us who don't like eating a big breakfast.

Most days I begin my day with a glass of water, feed the animals and birds, walk the dog, have my first cup of coffee, get all the humans set for the day—then around 9 or 10, I have another cup of coffee and some toast. Maybe half of a grapefruit if I'm missing my Uncle Ross—the only breakfast he ate: 1/2 grapefruit, 1/2 of an English muffin and coffee. I'm not sure if Uncle Ross was mindful or had OCD, but he lived a long healthy life.

What makes the difference in "just toast" is the quality of a toasted hunk of bread. I love making homemade bread but when I can't, or life gets too busy, the local grocery store carries a very nice variety. The phrase, "our daily bread" is a reminder for us to create and uphold a daily practice. We all choose for ourselves what that practice will be, mine is grounded in love and gratitude.

What can seem boring and mundane is the same thing that gives consistency through variety. In this case, bread is the constant though the type of bread may change.

There are so many toppings you can put on toast. The possibilities are endless. I love jams, jellies, peanut butter, smashed fresh fruit, or sprinkles of hemp or chia seeds to name a few. Avocado toast is also incredible! Love is the constant but how we live it each day offers unlimited possibilities.

Mantra: I am seeing myself as unlimited possibilities.

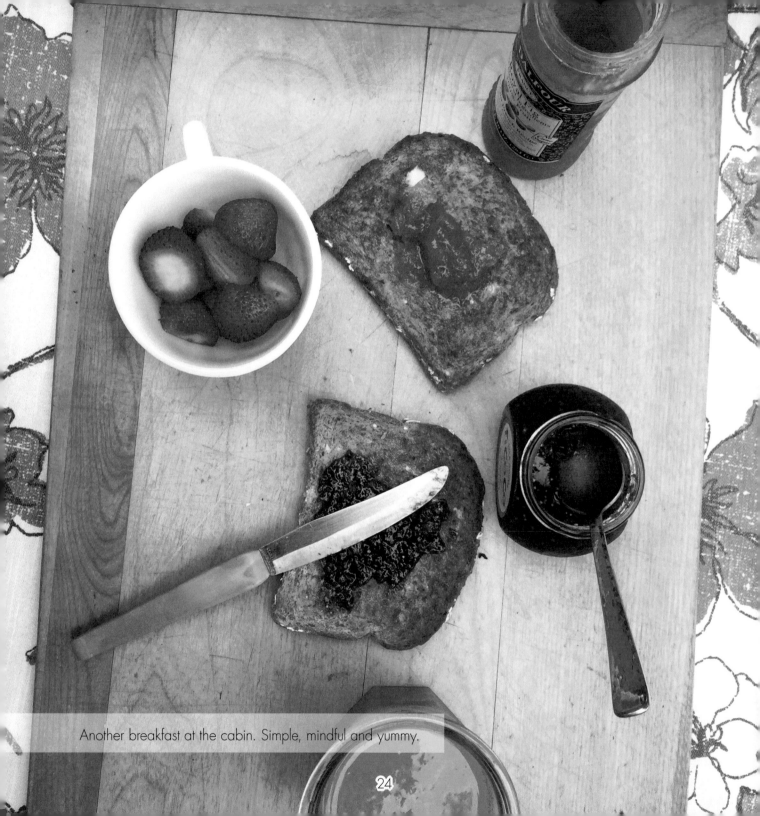

Another breakfast at the cabin. Simple, mindful and yummy.

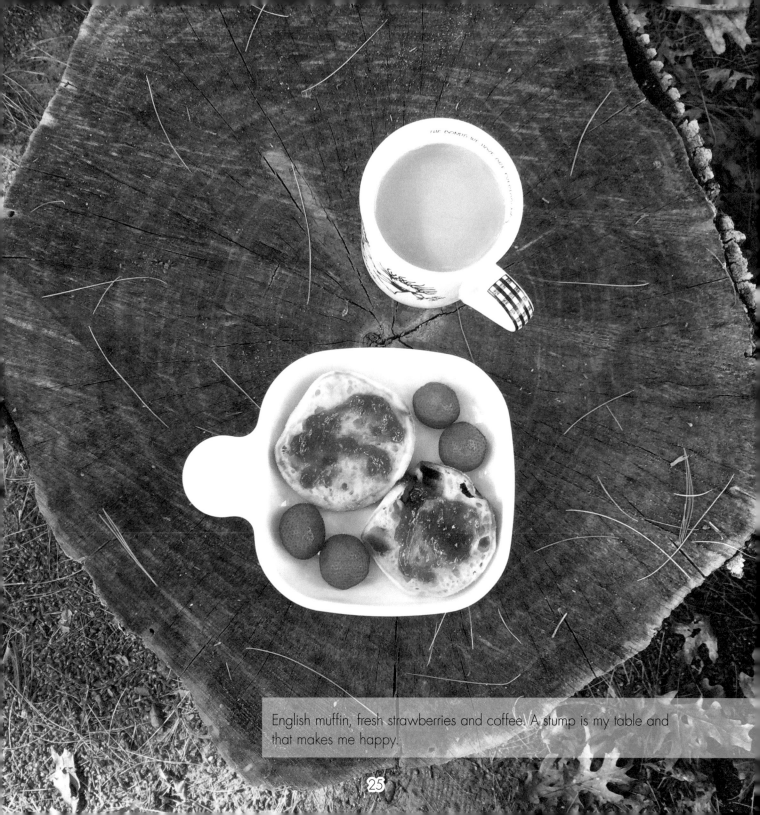

English muffin, fresh strawberries and coffee. A stump is my table and that makes me happy.

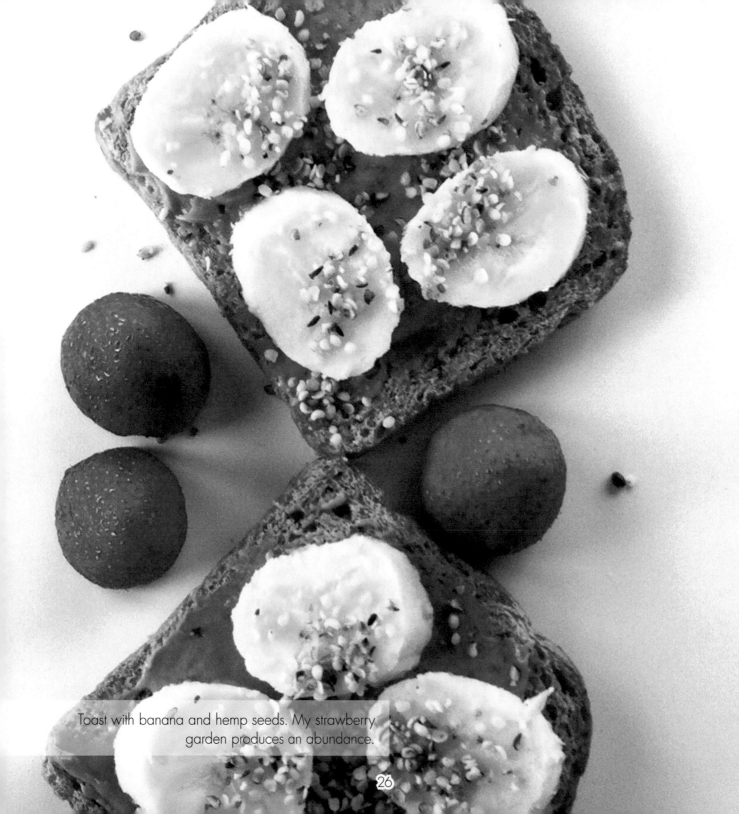

Toast with banana and hemp seeds. My strawberry garden produces an abundance.

BREAKFAST 2: GREEN SMOOTHIE

The on-the-go breakfast.

This green drink makes me feel radiant.

Banana, spinach, or dinosaur kale—the only kale I like—and orange juice. I also use Minute Maid Kids for the extra vitamins.

½ - 1 banana
A handful of greens
6 oz. of orange juice
Zoom it up in a blender and add ice.
It's that simple.

This is the only smoothie I like. I've tried 1000's of recipes—I'm not kidding. I've choked down some of the most God-awful concoctions, trusting foolishly what others wrote. But no. This is the smoothie I drink. I have tried adding a protein powder into it. It was okay, but I like it better without. When I first came across the green smoothie, I knew a green drink was going to be amazingly healthy; my mind said yes but my eyes said no thank you. It took some tweaking but now that I've found the perfect recipe for me, I wholeheartedly love the green smoothie. I'm so happy I can share this recipe with you too.

At the same time, I know people who like trying lots and lots of different smoothie recipes. I'm not one of them. I'm not adventurous when it involves my green drinks. I accept that about myself and others too (I have one kid who ate the same breakfast every day for years and another kid who doesn't want the same thing twice in a week). When we understand and accept ourselves, making choices becomes easier. When we stop trying to eat the way someone else suggests, we can settle in with what matters to us and just be ourselves.

Give yourself Green Smoothie grace. I believe in the importance of trying something new and I also honor my final choice.

Mantra: I welcome new opportunities and honor my final choice.

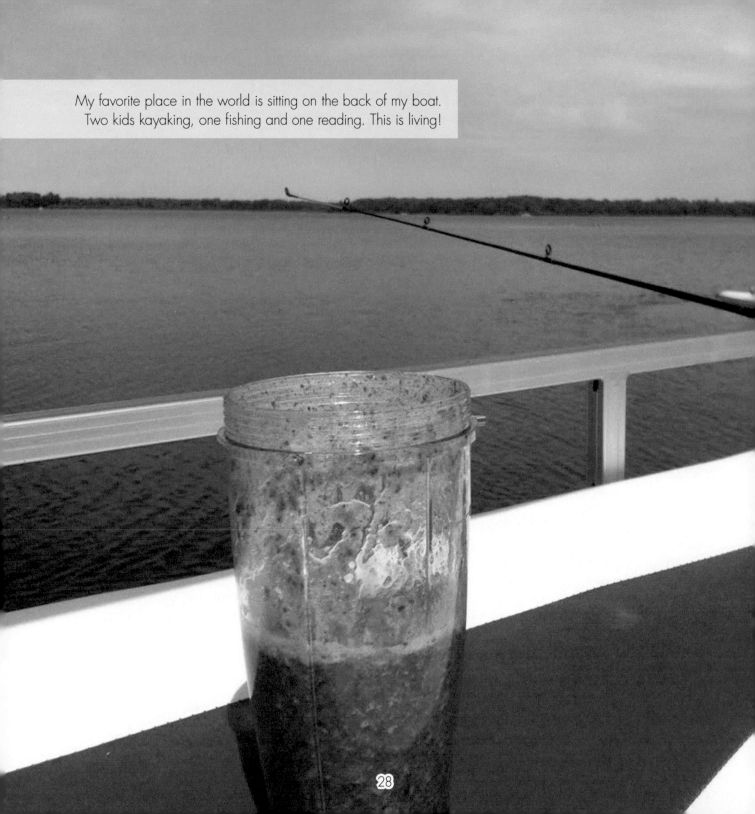

My favorite place in the world is sitting on the back of my boat.
Two kids kayaking, one fishing and one reading. This is living!

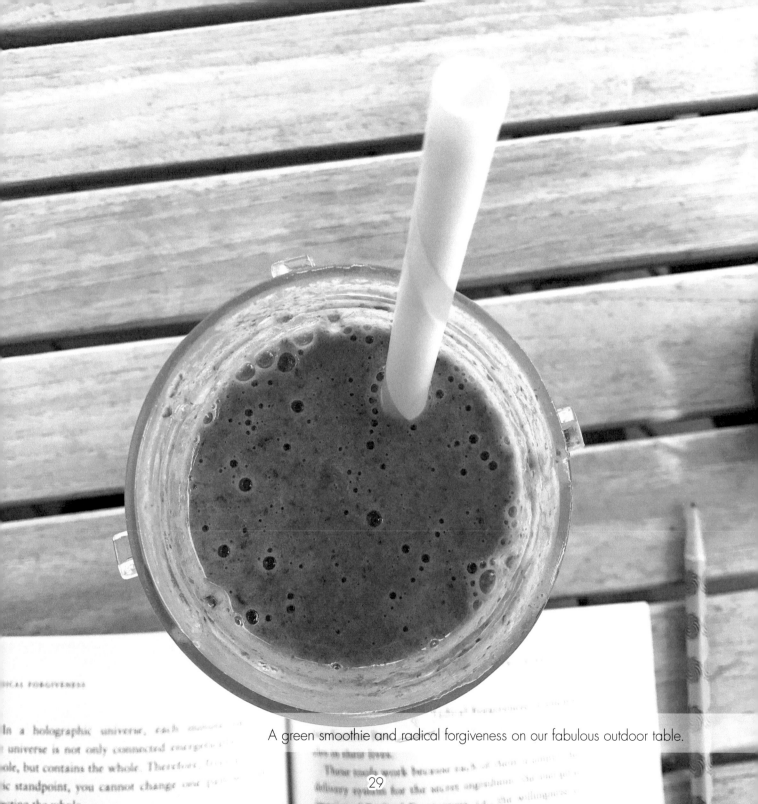

A green smoothie and radical forgiveness on our fabulous outdoor table.

BREAKFAST 3: GRANOLA

Sometimes straight out of the bag. No fuss, no muss. It's that simple.

My favorite is Love Crunch or Vicki's recipe from Ann Arbor Vegan Kitchen.

Sometimes I add wonderful, creamy, almond or flax milk. During the holidays festive eggnog inspired almond milks are also delightful.

Note: Before buying granola read the label. Not all granolas are vegan. I'd also say read the ingredient list, many products are vegan but processed in a facility that processes milk. Spoiler Alert: I'm not *that* vegan. I'm a mom trying to feed six people (not all vegan) and double or triple that on weekends . . . I do my best with the time and resources that I have.

Granola also makes a wonderful snack! Sweet, crunchy, and earthy. The typical hippie food with good reason, it connects us to the earth and open fields.

Mantra: I am connecting to the earth and honoring her resources.

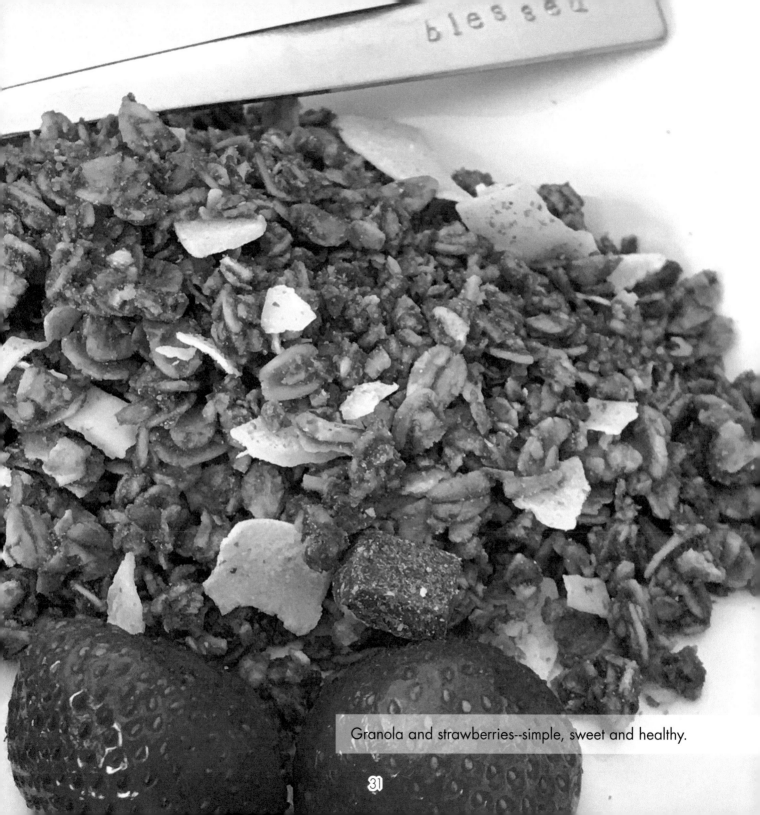

blessed

Granola and strawberries--simple, sweet and healthy.

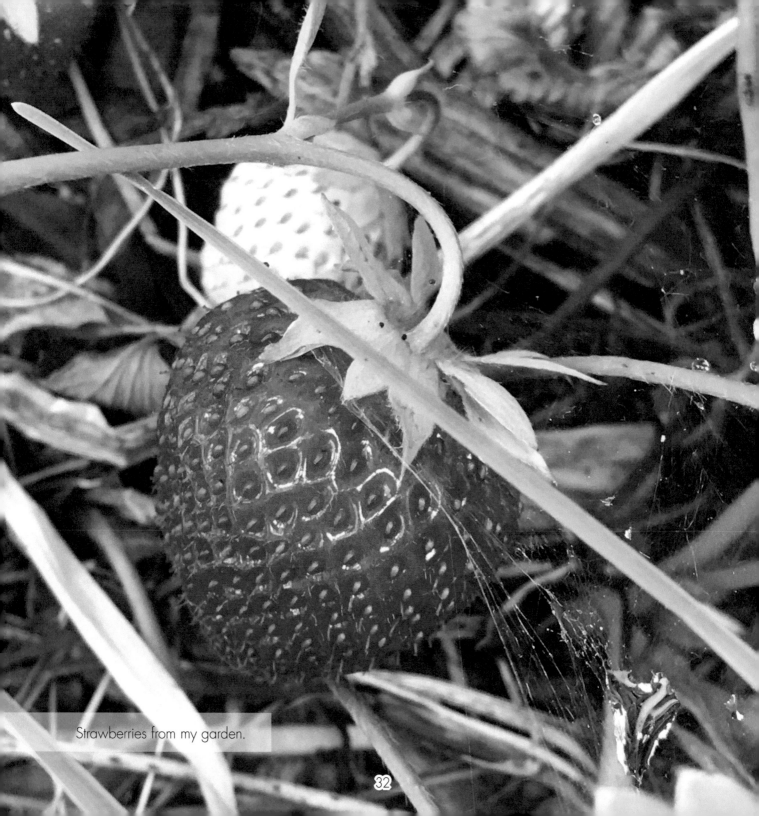

Strawberries from my garden.

BREAKFAST 4: MIXED VEGGIE EGGLESS FRITTATA

As a plant-based house, we always have lots of veggies in the fridge, and we usually have little bits of leftovers too. Maybe half an onion, two peppers, and one mini tree of broccoli. How I end up with all these bits is a mystery, but it happens.

I almost always have a bag of hash browns in the house too. They are inexpensive and easy to use in countless ways. This recipe honors the frugal part of my personality.

For a 10-inch skillet
1½ cups mixed veggies (peppers, onion, broccoli, mushrooms, etc.)
20 oz. bag of store bought hash browns
Olive oil or vegan spread
Salt and pepper to taste (cumin, red pepper flakes, fresh dill, or basil can also be nice additions)

Heat a skillet with a bit of olive oil or vegan spread specific to higher heat/sautéing

Add hash browns
Add raw veggies on top of hash browns. Cook until hash browns are crunchy on the bottom (this takes longer than you think, don't rush the potatoes!).
Flip the frittata until the raw veggies are cooked to your desired crunch.

As the hash browns cook, they will create lots of steam which cooks the veggies on top. You could cover them, but the hash browns won't be as crunchy on the bottom. It may take a few tries to figure out how you like this dish. This dish can NOT be rushed. It takes a bit of time but worth it.

Kitchen note: The pan makes all the difference when making hash browns—a yummy trial and error experiment. I use a cast iron pan that cooks the hash browns to a nice crunch while holding the heat.

Mantra: I am patient.

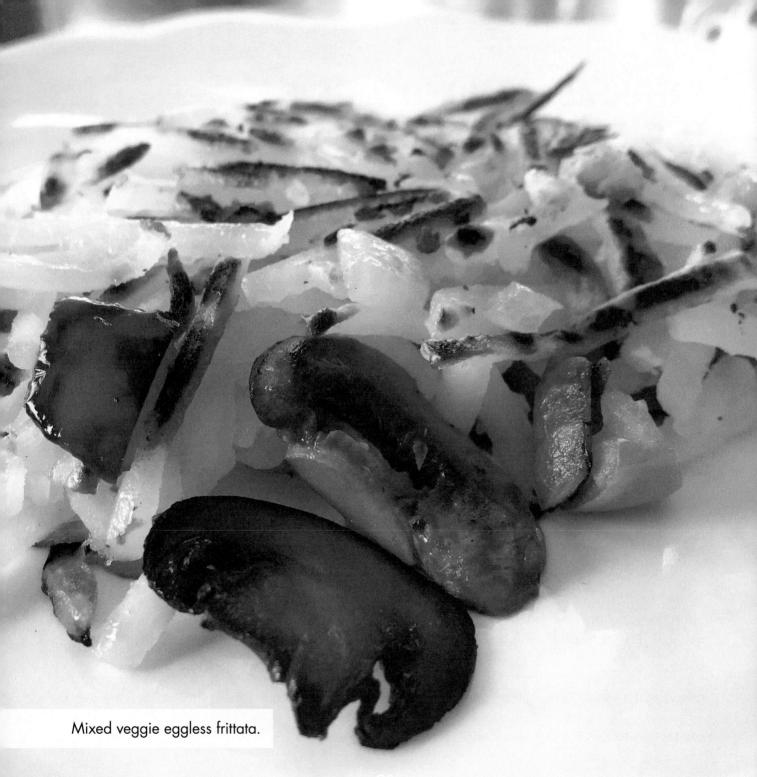

Mixed veggie eggless frittata.

BREAKFAST 5: OATMEAL

"I hate oatmeal," is something I've heard a lot. However, with so many different oatmeal options I believe there is something for everyone. But resistance can be difficult to overcome. We can dig our heels in deeper or we can choose to take the first step.

In his poem, *Sarah Cynthia Silvia Stout*, Shel Silverstein described it as "gloppy glumps of cold oatmeal." But oatmeal does not have to be gloppy, mushy, or gross. Not at all.

I make a 50/50 mix of oatmeal and muesli. It is a nutty, seedy, dried fruity blend of wonderfulness in a bowl.

Stove top directions:
1 cup of boiling water
½ cup 50/50 blend
Let boil 1 minute, turn heat down to simmer and cook 4 minutes
Take off heat, cover and let it sit for 2 minutes

Almost every Tuesday morning I make oatmeal. Everyone knows it will be warm and ready when they come to the kitchen. I top it with in-season fresh fruit, or my kitchen mainstay, the organic banana.
Add Michigan maple syrup.
Hemp seeds.
Cook it in almond milk vs. water. Or, cook it in the eggnog almond milk (Wouldn't that be phenomenal?).
This morning, while you prepare your oatmeal, begin your mindfulness practice:
Will you choose to be open or closed? To move towards love or fear?

Mantra: I am mindful of every choice I make.

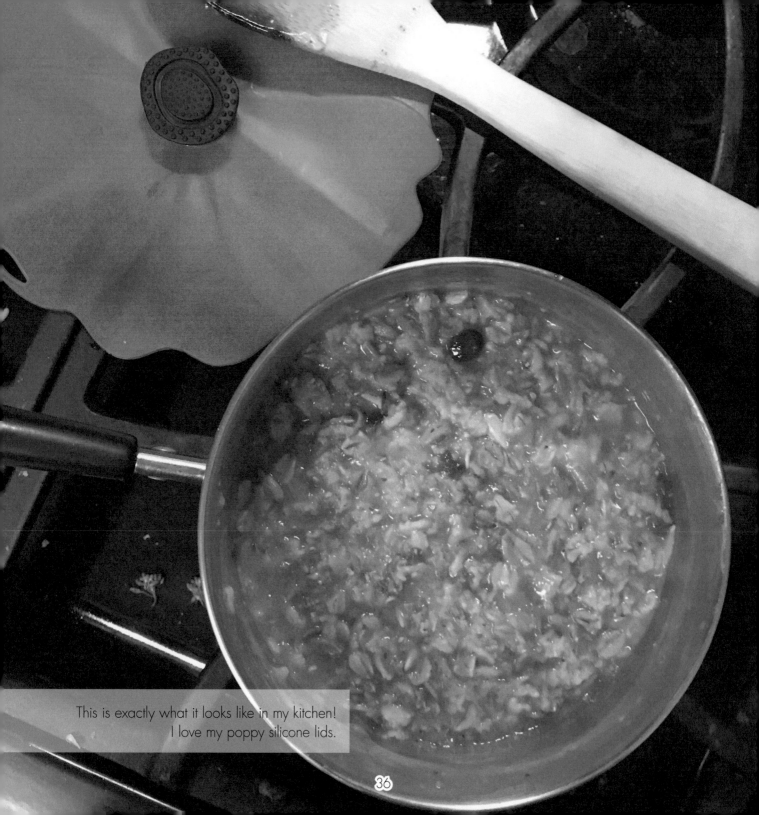

This is exactly what it looks like in my kitchen!
I love my poppy silicone lids.

36

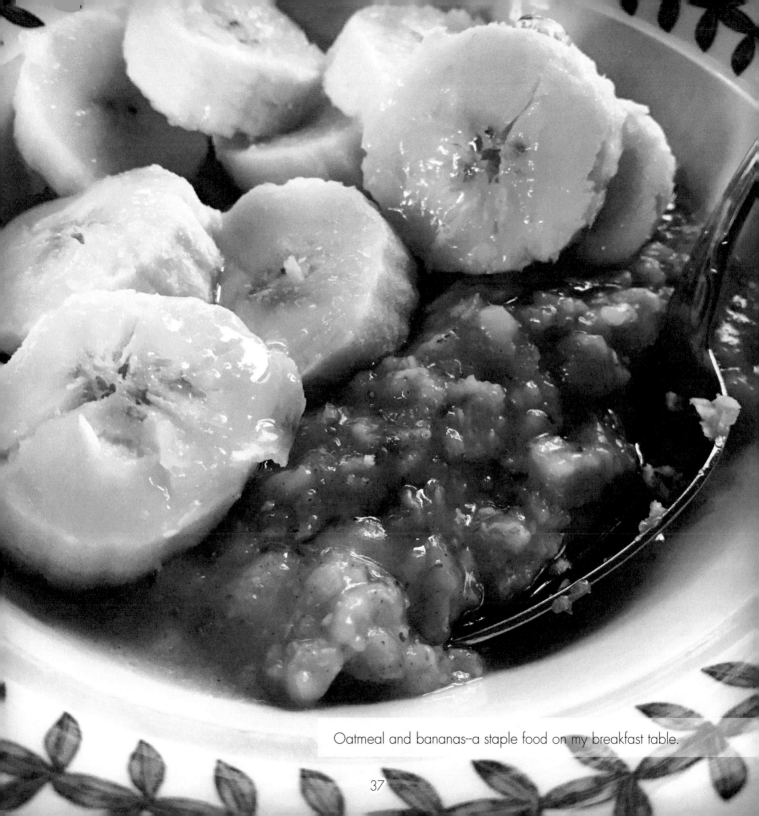

Oatmeal and bananas–a staple food on my breakfast table.

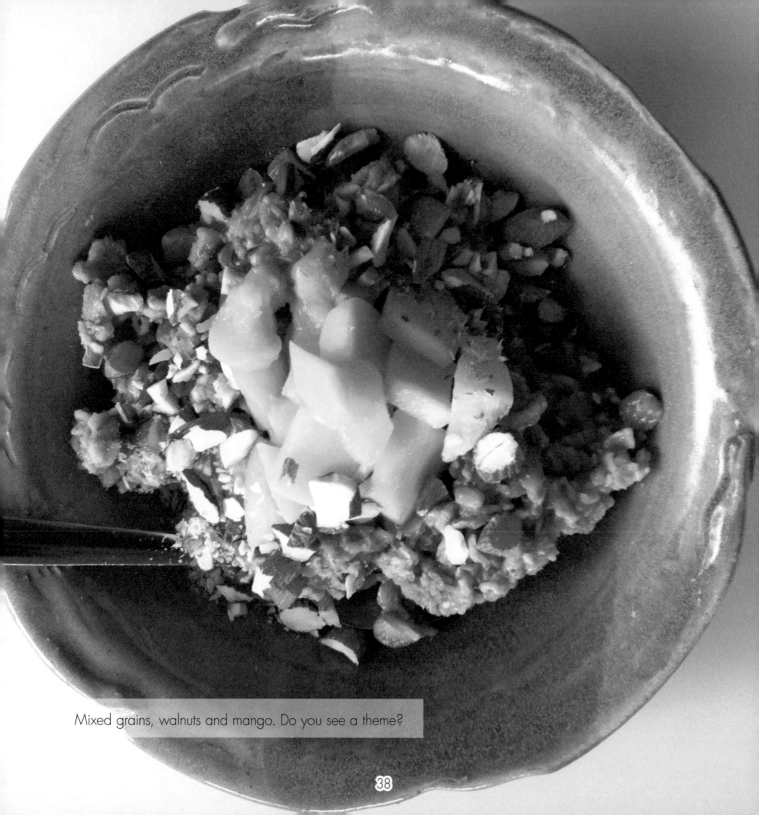

Mixed grains, walnuts and mango. Do you see a theme?

BREAKFAST 6: MAKE AHEAD CHIA PUDDING

Did you know the word chia is the Mayan word for strength? Who doesn't want to start their day strong? I've been making chia pudding for a very long time. The versatility of chia is beautiful. You can take any vegan beverage and make the pudding: chocolate almond milk, vanilla soy milk, the vegan eggnog . . . I've even used my green smoothie. The possibilities are endless.

Chia seeds are a tiny superfood! Loaded with heart-healthy Omega fatty acids, fiber, calcium, zinc, iron, and protein, and so versatile, you can sprinkle on just about any breakfast. My original recipe is shared here:

3 tbsp chia seeds
1 cup of almond milk (or whatever you chose to use),
Put ingredients it in a mason jar and shake.
The seeds will float.
Shake jar (4 good shakes) every 5 minutes for the first 20 minutes so seeds don't clump together.
Refrigerate until firm.

Chia pudding bowls are very and easy and very tasty. Simply make the pudding, then add fruit, granola, and whatever your imagination can come up with. This type of cookbook allows you, begs you, to come up with your own ideas.

Chia seeds are the tiniest seed I've ever seen. They grow and expand tremendously. Each day we grow and expand in mind, body and spirit, why not tune into that process?

Mantra: I am transforming.

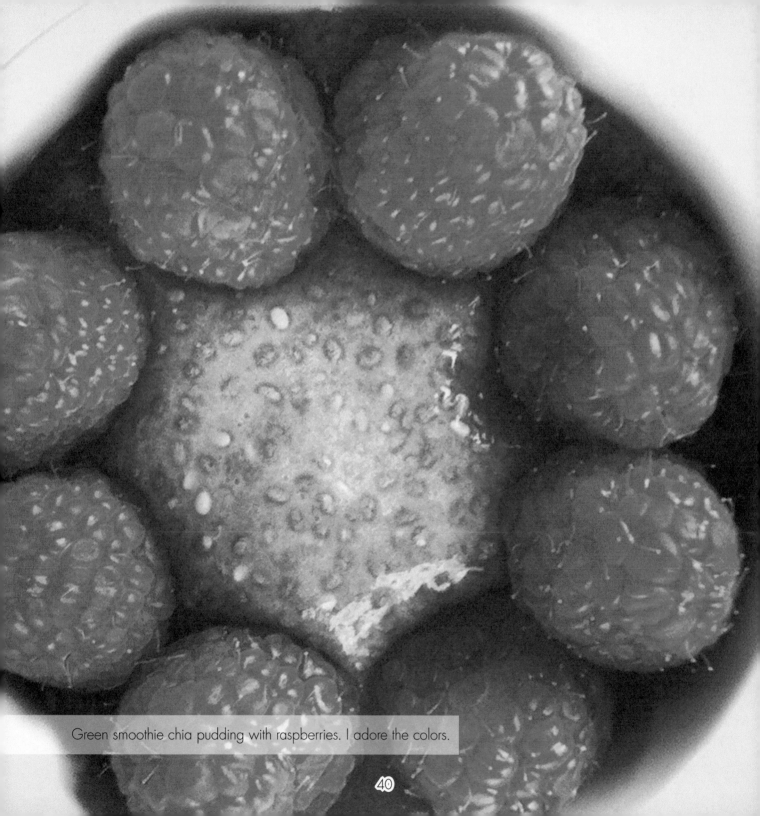

Green smoothie chia pudding with raspberries. I adore the colors.

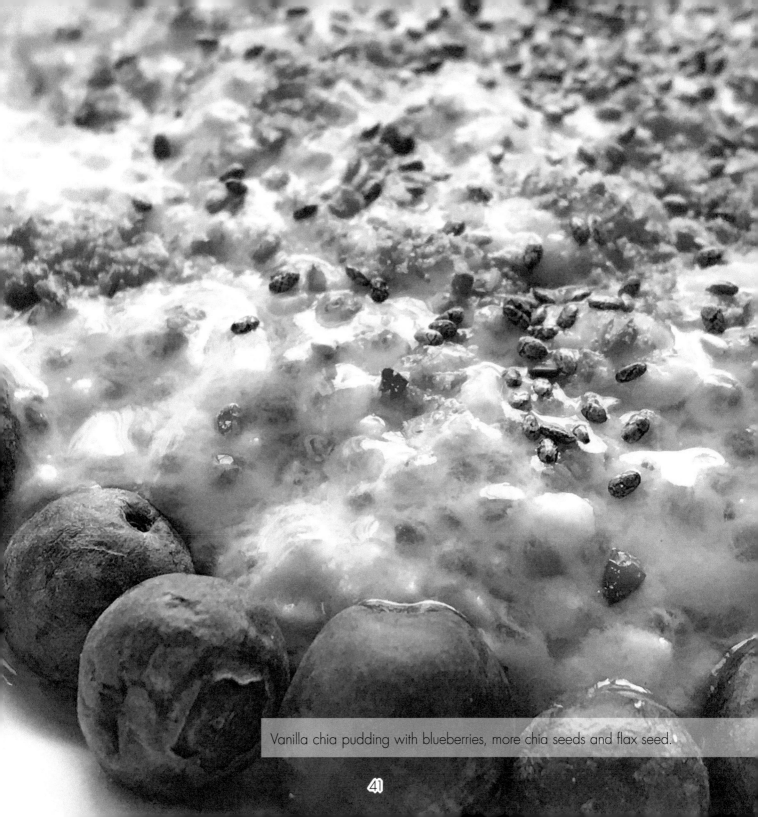

Vanilla chia pudding with blueberries, more chia seeds and flax seed.

BREAKFAST 7: GRAINS BREAKFAST BOWL

A grains bowl is a texture explosion in your mouth.

On weeks I want to have a grains bowl breakfast I will make quinoa, add leftover rice or barley, and then add oatmeal or an oatmeal pouch that has a few different grains included.

I like the Think Thin brand and Elizabeth brands. I may add hemp seeds or chia seeds. It is very much a hodgepodge of using leftovers for breakfast. It can be sweet or savory. I prefer sweet! I also like adding fruit, dark sweet cherries are my favorite.

I realize this is more of a recipe *idea* and not a recipe. But exact, measured out recipes isn't how I roll. Nature produces, and we get creative. That is what this cookbook is all about.

In theory, it should be easy to be gentle, loving, kind, and respectful in life, but it is not. We need to be committed to trying each day. Life isn't always calculated and planned like a recipe, instead it is often a spontaneous, unpredictable adventure.

Mantra: I am committed to trying every day to be the best version of myself knowing that some days will be harder than others.

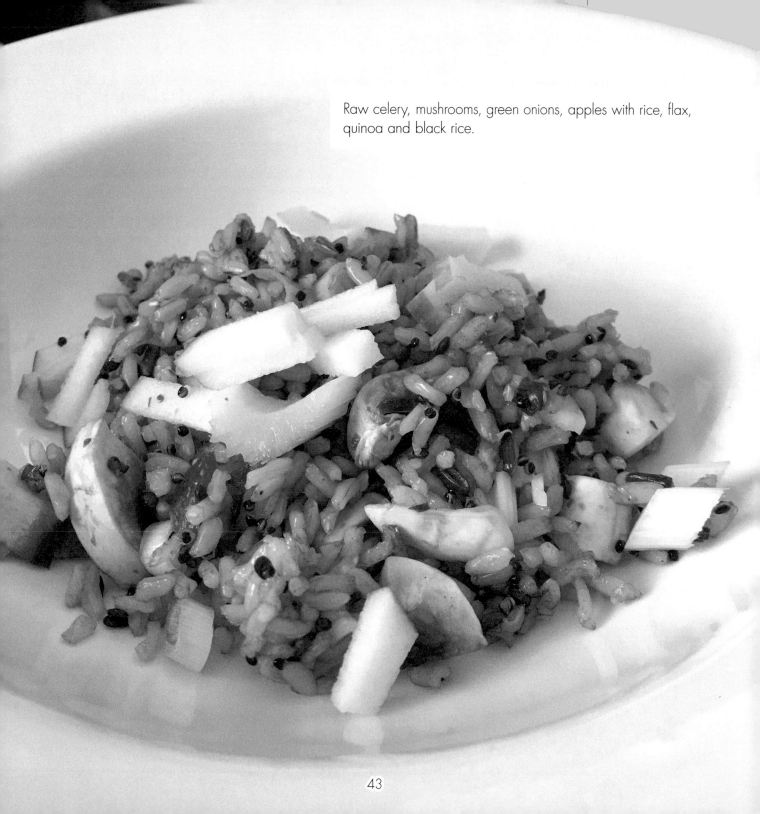

Raw celery, mushrooms, green onions, apples with rice, flax, quinoa and black rice.

BREAKFAST 8: WAFFLE BANANA SANDWICH

I ate this sandwich almost every day during two of my pregnancies. It was quick, easy, and it filled me up. It is also a great on the go breakfast for one of my kids who is chronically late.

My favorite: Figs, walnuts, bananas, creamy peanut butter on a warm, crunchy waffle.

Super simple: Vegan waffle slathered with vegan peanut butter and ½ of a smashed banana.

Food does not need to be complicated. Keep it simple. In fact, often, the simpler, the healthier.

I hope everyone will be as excited as I am about food and being mindful of our relationships with each other—the earth and all living things. Honestly, I have my moments of getting overwhelmed. When I'm not gentle, loving, kind, or respectful—I try to recognize it, accept what the situation is, investigate with kindness, and allow natural awareness to present itself.

Mantra: I embrace simple.

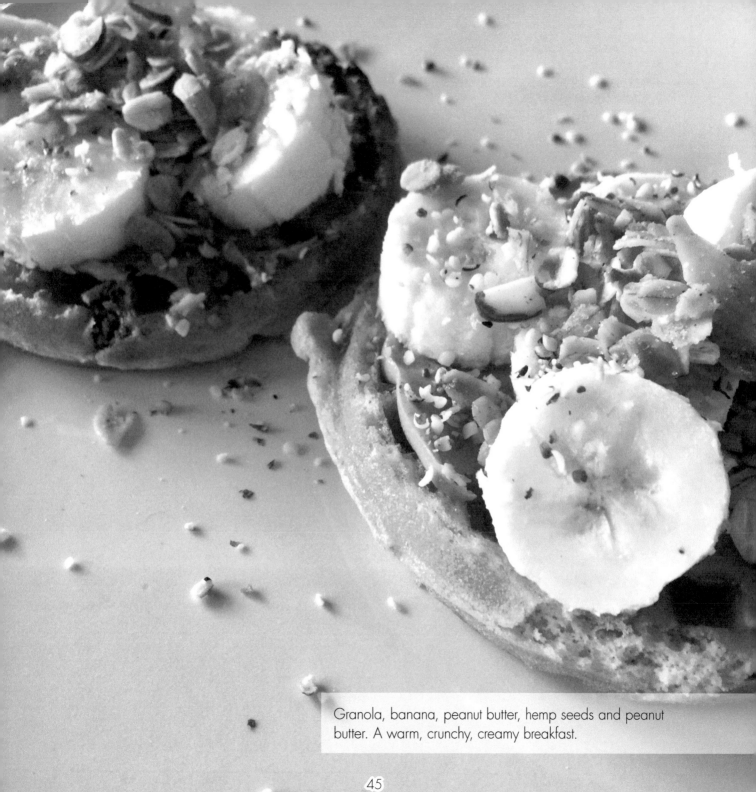

Granola, banana, peanut butter, hemp seeds and peanut butter. A warm, crunchy, creamy breakfast.

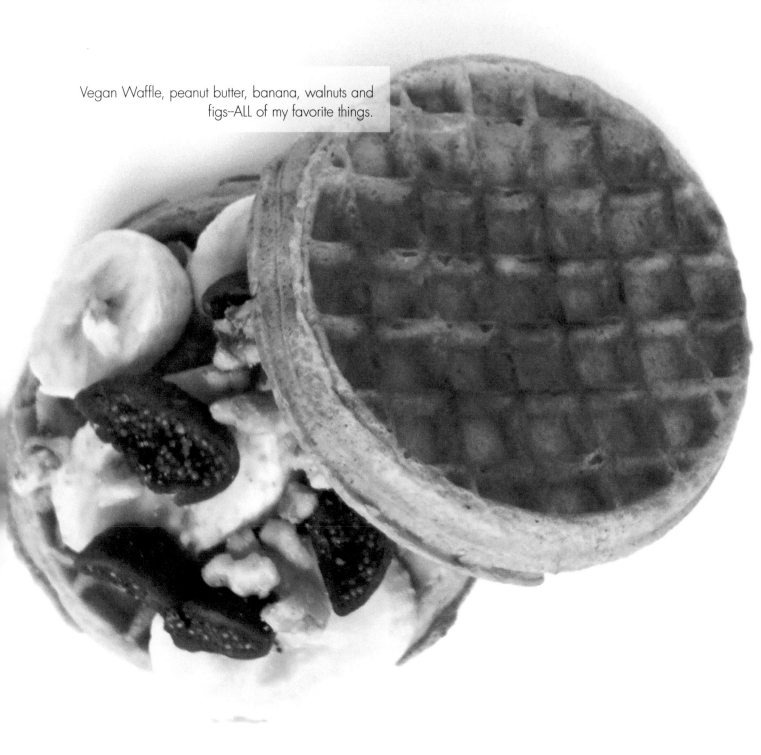

Vegan Waffle, peanut butter, banana, walnuts and figs--ALL of my favorite things.

BREAKFAST 9: PANCAKES TO DIE FOR!!!

Nearly every Sunday morning I make a pancake breakfast for my family. It is a tradition I stumbled into when the kids were toddlers. Now, every Saturday night sleepover my kids and their friends will have the Sunday morning welcomed with pancakes. I think it is a marvelous legacy to have.

1 cup flour
¾ cup of milk substitute. I use almond milk eggnog.
1 tbsp baking powder
½ tsp salt
3 tbsp maple syrup or agave
Mix the dry ingredients first then add the milk and the agave/syrup. If the mix is too thick, add more liquid.

The amount of liquid can vary. The first time I made these I used ¾ cup almond milk and the second time I used 1 cup eggnog flavored coconut milk.

I cook the pancakes in a cast iron skillet with vegan spread. They are fluffy yet crisp— heavenly.

Sometimes I add organic wild blueberries from Trader Joe's—the tiny berries remind me of picking "blues," the nickname for blueberries, on the shores of Lake Superior.

This is my go-to pancake mix. The kids love it, and it is a small batch which gives me enough time to make weekday morning pancakes for the kids.

Mantra: I am thankful for the sun, water, wind, and earth working in harmony to create beautiful ingredients to nourish our bodies and delight our souls.

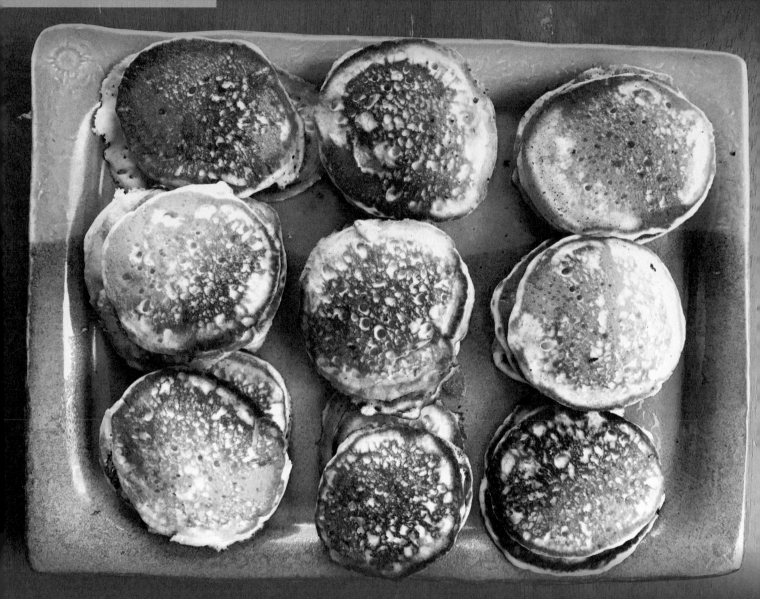

Pancakes for my family.

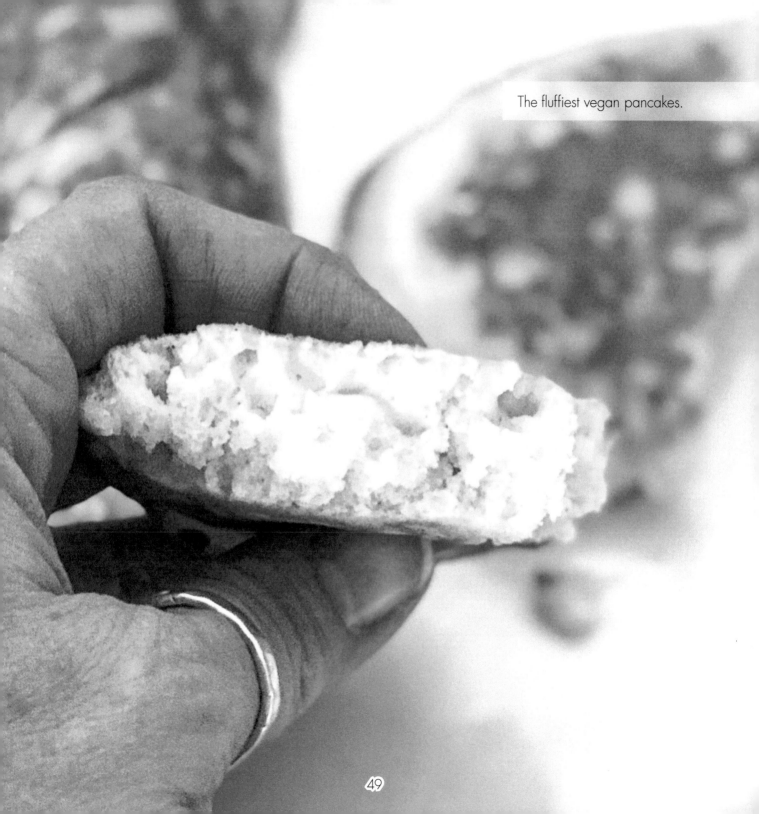

The fluffiest vegan pancakes.

BREAKFAST 10: FRUIT BOWL WITH GRANOLA AND VEGAN YOGURT PARFAIT

I make a yogurt parfait that looks pretty, is fun to eat and I can make ahead. I add the granola right before I serve it.

The versatility of this breakfast is unlimited. Change the fruit, switch up the yogurt, use granola, chia pudding, or oatmeal. The possibilities are endless.

Mantra: My life is like a parfait, layered with wonderfulness.

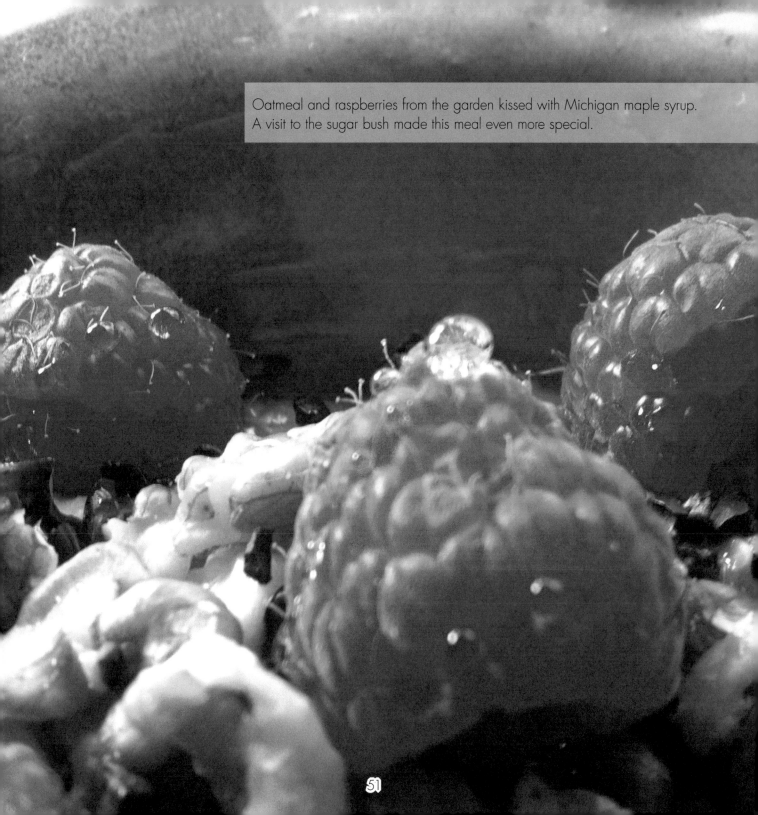

Oatmeal and raspberries from the garden kissed with Michigan maple syrup.
A visit to the sugar bush made this meal even more special.

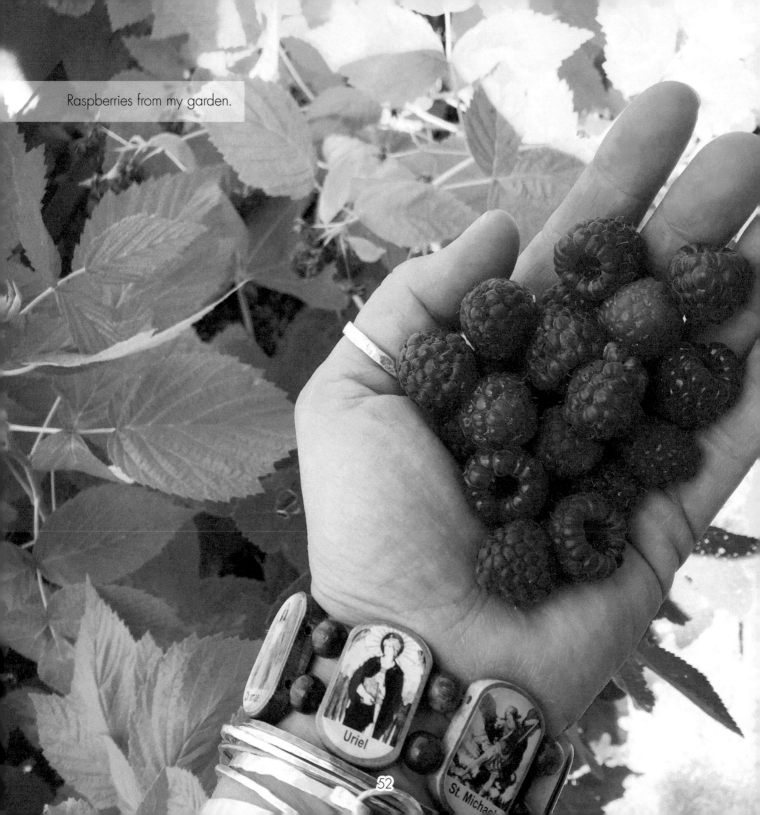

Raspberries from my garden.

52

PLANT BASED MADE SUPER EASY

It is easy for you to be blessed by your breakfast. How wonderful to begin your day honoring your body, the earth, and the animals. To begin to think about where your food is coming from, how it was grown, who picked it . . . who put it on the shelves at the store? Who is cooking it?

You are a beautiful divine being.

Say that out loud with me: "I am a beautiful divine being."

When you feel that in your bones (it may take time, but that's okay!); you will begin to see the beauty in everything and everyone. We become one but not the same. Do not confuse oneness with sameness. Think of yourself as a passing dish at a potluck. You bring your best version of you, which is totally different than my best version of me, and together we create a beautiful banquet.

When we begin our practice of morning mindfulness, being blessed by breakfast, we begin a journey to become the best version of ourselves. We continue our practice one mindful moment at a time, throughout the day, the week, the month, and the years. Life is cumulative. We may have mindful moments infrequently BUT as you increase your awareness and desire to be mindful they will increase. We choose mindfulness.

We chose to be blessed by breakfast.

We choose to find our truth.

We choose to see ourselves as worthy.

Loved.

Heard.

Nourished.

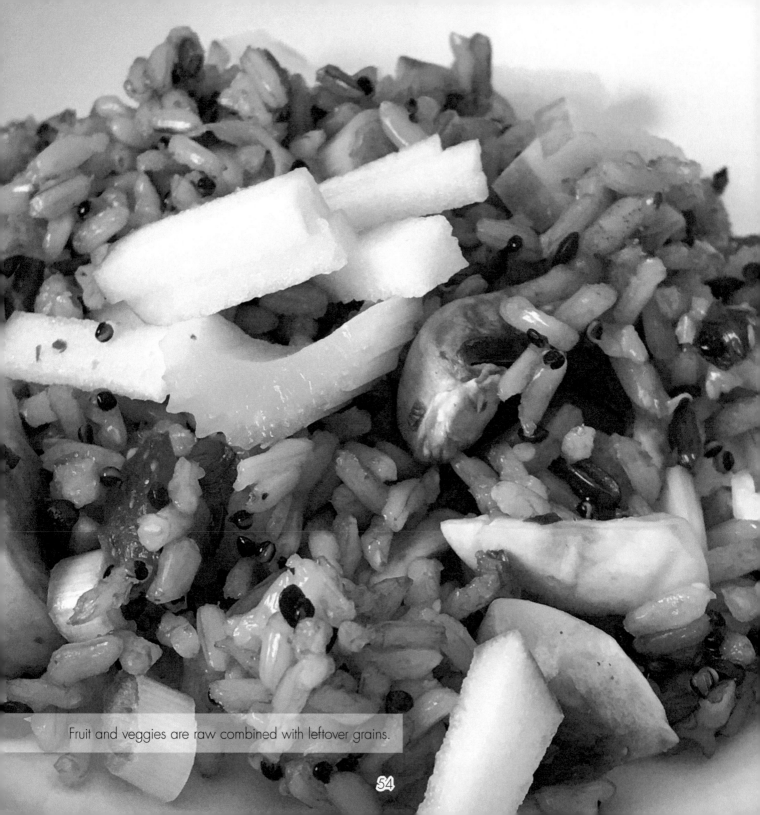

Fruit and veggies are raw combined with leftover grains.

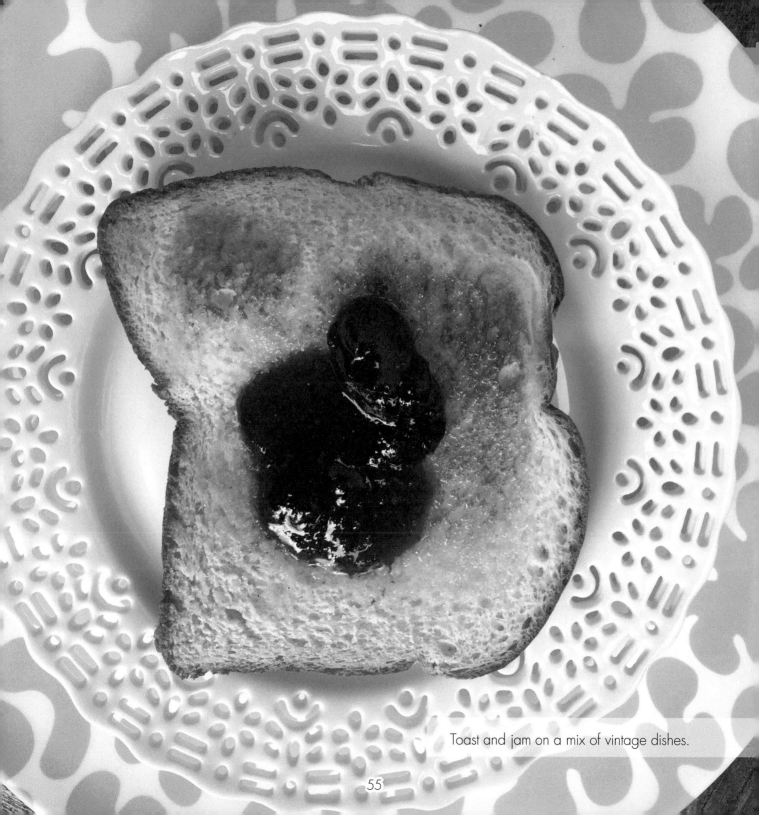

Toast and jam on a mix of vintage dishes.

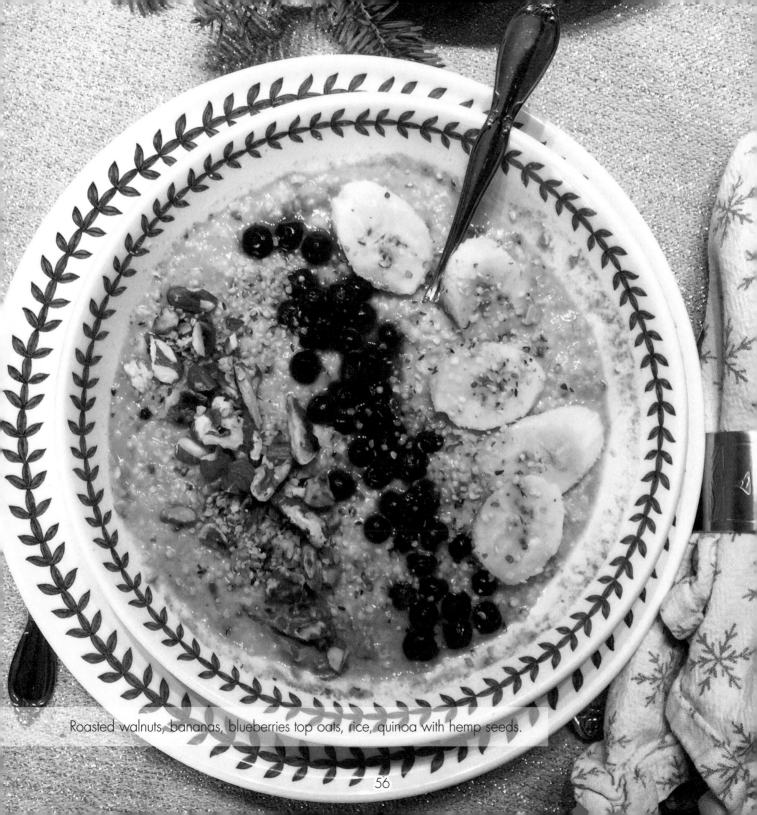

Roasted walnuts, bananas, blueberries top oats, rice, quinoa with hemp seeds.

Acknowledgments

I'd like to thank everyone on my team; everyone who loves me and supports me. You know who you are because I tell you all the time. I love you and adore you.

Teddy Roosevelt for this quote and Brene Brown for bringing it to my attention:

"It is not the critic who counts; not the man who points out how the strong man stumbles, or where the doer of deeds could have done them better. The credit belongs to the man who is actually in the arena, whose face is marred by dust and sweat and blood; who strives valiantly; who errs, who comes short again and again, because there is no effort without error and shortcoming; but who does actually strive to do the deeds; who knows great enthusiasms, the great devotions; who spends himself in a worthy cause; who at the best knows in the end the triumph of high achievement, and who at the worst, if he fails, at least fails while daring greatly, so that his place shall never be with those cold and timid souls who neither know victory nor defeat."

Seth Godin for your inspiring words "Renée, just keep making a ruckus!"

The conversations that I have had with Gene Baur have inspired me to find my voice and speak from the heart.

The honor of Gene Stone reading over my manuscript, three years after our first emails. Divine timing. Thank you for your comments and blessing.

Thanks to Stacey and Kay for your editorial genius. A special thanks to Frank for just being there 24/7 offering inspiration.

To the sisterhood that supports me when I ask for help and probably more importantly when I don't-- they know how to give from the heart just when I need it most.

To my brother who eats anything and everything that I make.

I am most thankful and appreciative for Eric and my four kids. Being a wife and a mother is the only thing I have ever wanted to be . . . thank you.

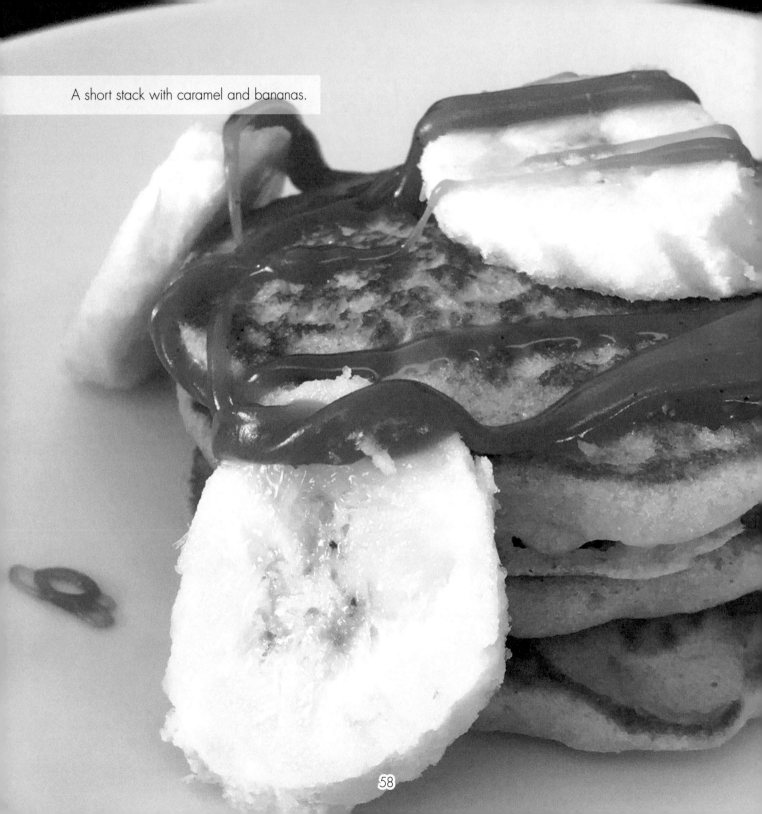

A short stack with caramel and bananas.

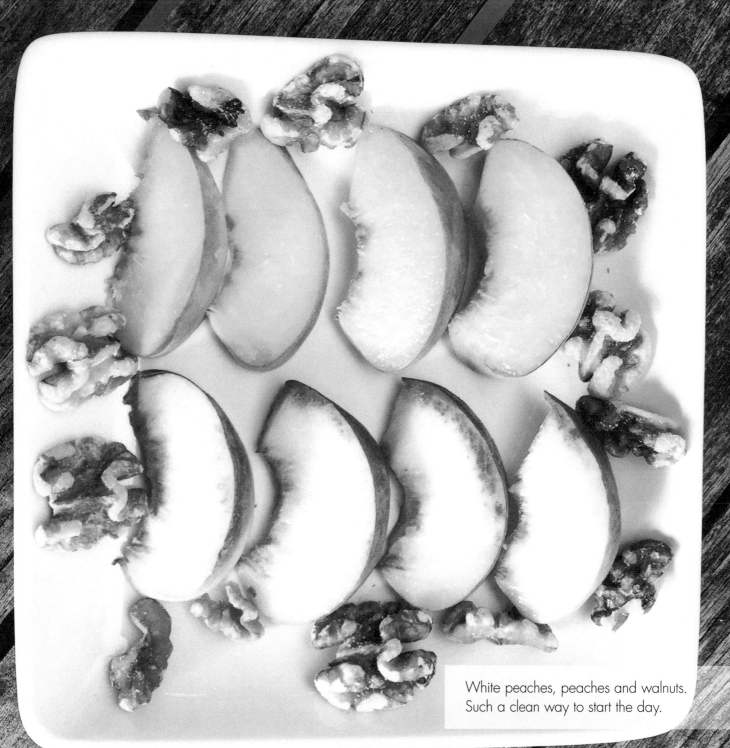

White peaches, peaches and walnuts.
Such a clean way to start the day.

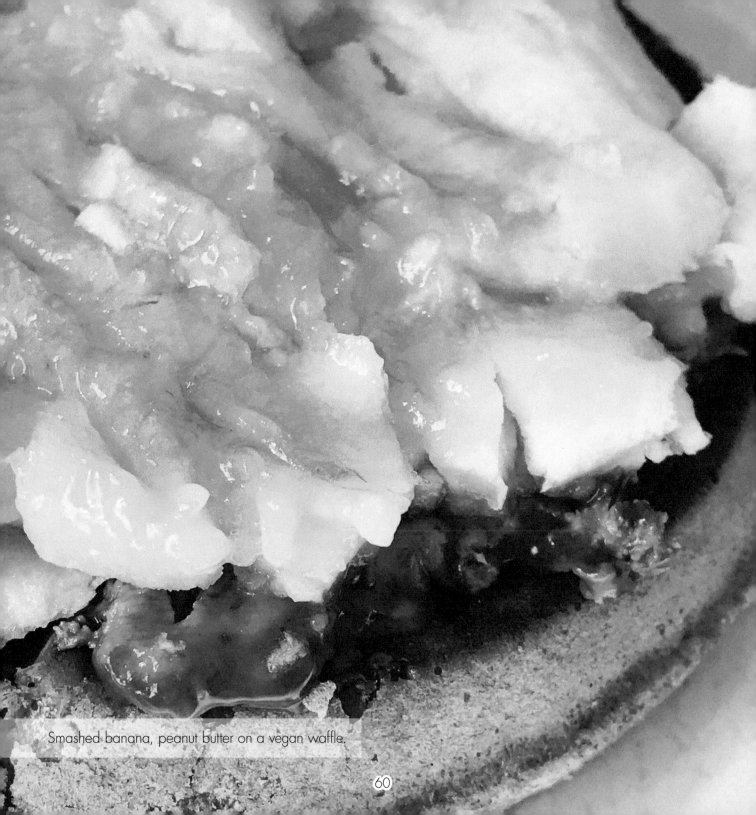

Smashed banana, peanut butter on a vegan waffle.

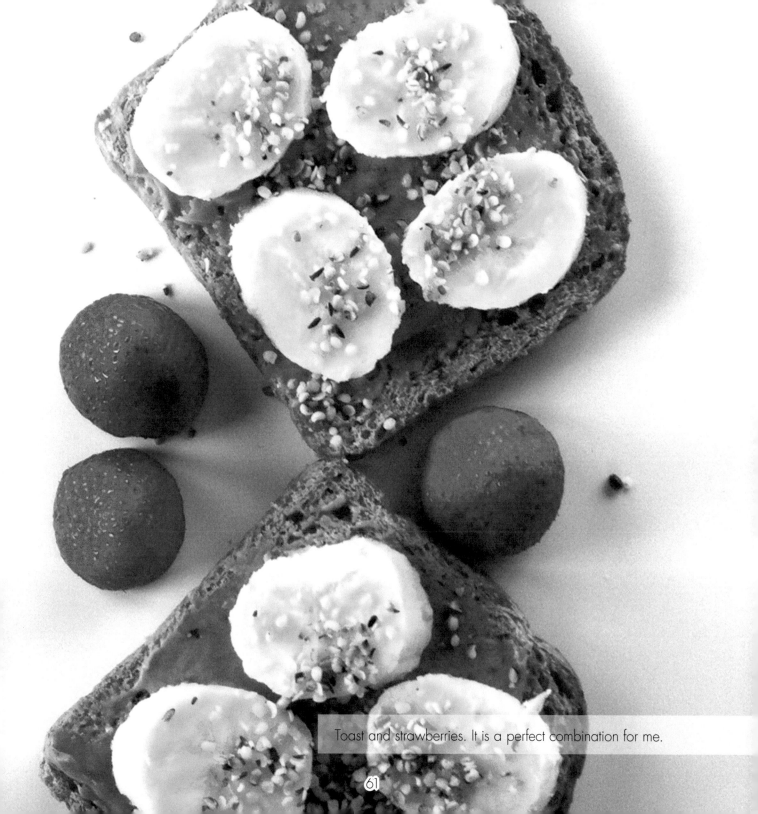

Toast and strawberries. It is a perfect combination for me.

61

Printed in the United States
By Bookmasters